THE HUMAN BODY IN 3D

THE HEAD AND NECK IN 3D

rosen publishing's
rosen central®

JACINTHA NATHAN
AND WALTER OLEKSY

Published in 2016 by The Rosen Publishing Group, Inc.
29 East 21st Street, New York, NY 10010

First Edition

Library of Congress Cataloging-in-Publication Data

Nathan, Jacintha.
The head and neck in 3D/Jacintha Nathan and Walter Oleksy.—First edition.
   pages cm.—(The human body in 3D)
Includes bibliographical references and index.
ISBN 978-1-4994-3593-1 (library bound)—ISBN 978-1-4994-3595-5 (pbk.)—
ISBN 978-1-4994-3596-2 (6-pack)
1. Head—Anatomy—Juvenile literature. 2. Neck—Anatomy—Juvenile literature. I. Oleksy, Walter G., 1930- II. Title.
QM535.N38 2016
612.9'1—dc23
                                                           2015000224

Manufactured in the United States of America

CONTENTS

INTRODUCTION

The shape of the head and neck comes from the bones of the skull and upper spinal column. The bones of the skull give shape to the human face, possibly the area most focused on in the entire body. The head and neck house the brain and brain stem, as well as nerves, the command center of the body, without which a person could not function. The skull and muscles of the head also house the eyes, ears, nose, mouth, teeth, tongue, and throat. They control a person's ability to see, hear, smell, taste, eat, and speak. This area of the body is a focus of study by many professionals, from neuroscientists to speech pathologists.

For much of human history, the function of the brain in particular remained a mystery. It was the Greek physician and philosopher Galen (129–c. 216 CE) who first recognized the brain, rather than the heart, as the center of human activity. He also discovered that the larynx was responsible for generating the voice. Owing to his diligent study of animals, Galen's medical abilities were quite advanced for his time. His method of removing cataracts from the eye mirrors a modern approach.

The head and neck house complex systems comprising bone, soft tissue, and organs.

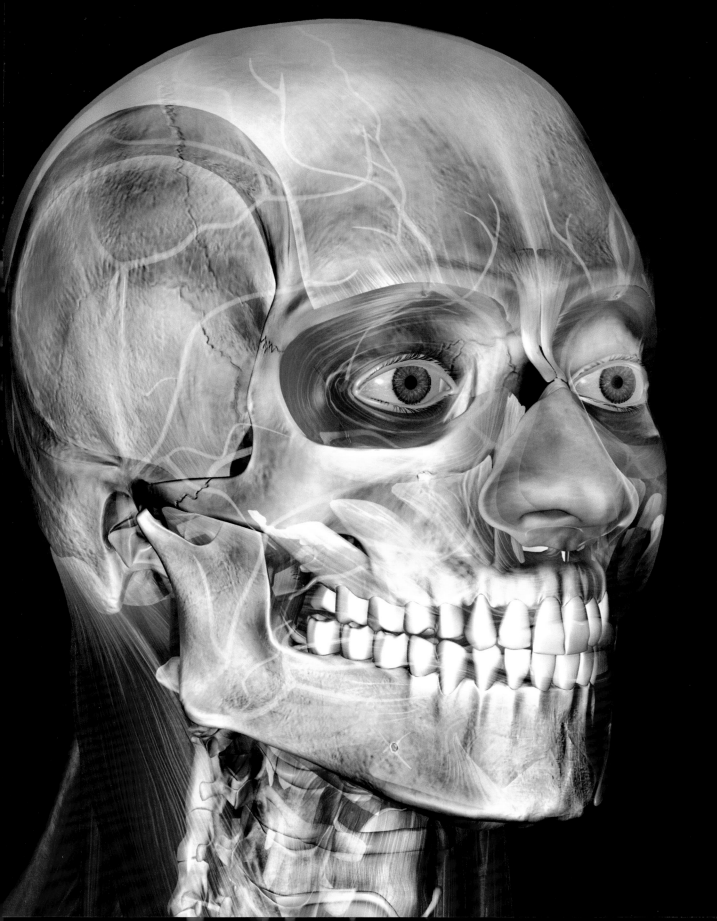

Both legitimate scientific study and pseudoscience have made several blunders regarding the functioning and treatment of the brain. Phrenology, from the Greek *phren* ("mind") and *logos* ("knowledge") was popular in the nineteenth century. This combination of neuroanatomy and philosophy was developed by German physician Franz Joseph Gall in the 1700s. He assumed that a person's character and thoughts were governed by the physical shape of the person's head. He developed the method of measuring and feeling a person's skull to determine his or her psychological traits. Phrenology was used to explain criminal behavior as well as show European superiority over other races.

The study of psychology, in attempts to heal mental illness, relied on sometimes violent and cruel methods. People who were mentally ill were once thought to be possessed by demons, so a hole was cut into the skull in order to let the demons out. In the seventeenth and eighteenth centuries, people were tortured in an attempt to change their thinking. Psychosurgery involved destroying parts of the brain, which left patients with permanent brain damage that affected their ability to live normal lives afterward. In the eighteenth century, French physician Philippe Pinel called for more moderate restraints at a Paris asylum and found that the patients were thereafter more responsive to treatment. He advocated for individual treatment, creating case files for patients, and attempted to find different types of treatment for different types of mental disorders. However, brutal methods continued into the twentieth century, and electroshock therapy is still used as a last resort today. Despite many modern advances, medical scientists still have not unlocked all of the brain's functions, so neuroscience is still heavily studied.

Although the brain is easily the most studied part of the body, the head and neck house other parts vital to the function of the human body. ENTs focus on the functioning of the ear, nose, and throat; ophthalmologists study the health and function of the eye and optic nerves; speech pathologists focus on the mouth, tongue, and throat; dentists concentrate on tooth and gum health. These are just a few of the medical professions that are dedicated to the study of the head and neck.

CHAPTER ONE

BONES OF THE HEAD AND NECK

The skeleton provides internal support to the body and surrounds and protects soft organs such as the brain. An adult skeleton has 206 bones, which connect at joints and move freely. The skeleton also consists of cartilage and ligaments. The flexible tissue that forms the framework of the ear and nose, for example, is made of cartilage. Ligaments are strong connective tissue that hold bones together at the joints. There are more than six hundred skeletal muscles, which are attached to the bones. Muscles hold the skeleton together and facilitate movement.

Bones are a type of connective tissue that has a rich supply of blood, lymph vessels, and nerves. Although they look fragile, bones are as strong as cast iron but much lighter, with a degree of flexibility that allows them to withstand forces of movement. All bones are surrounded by connective tissue. This outer layer, called the periosteum, contains cells that help

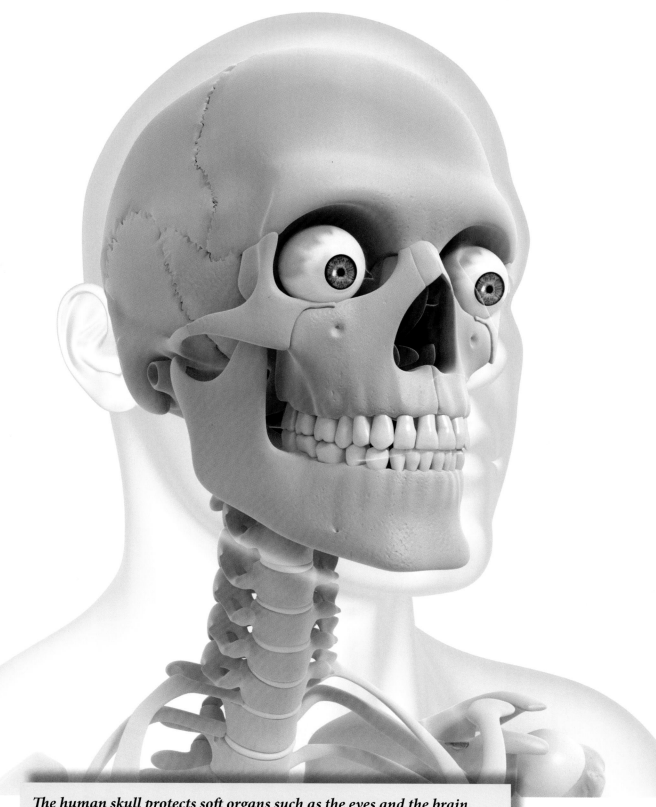

The human skull protects soft organs such as the eyes and the brain.

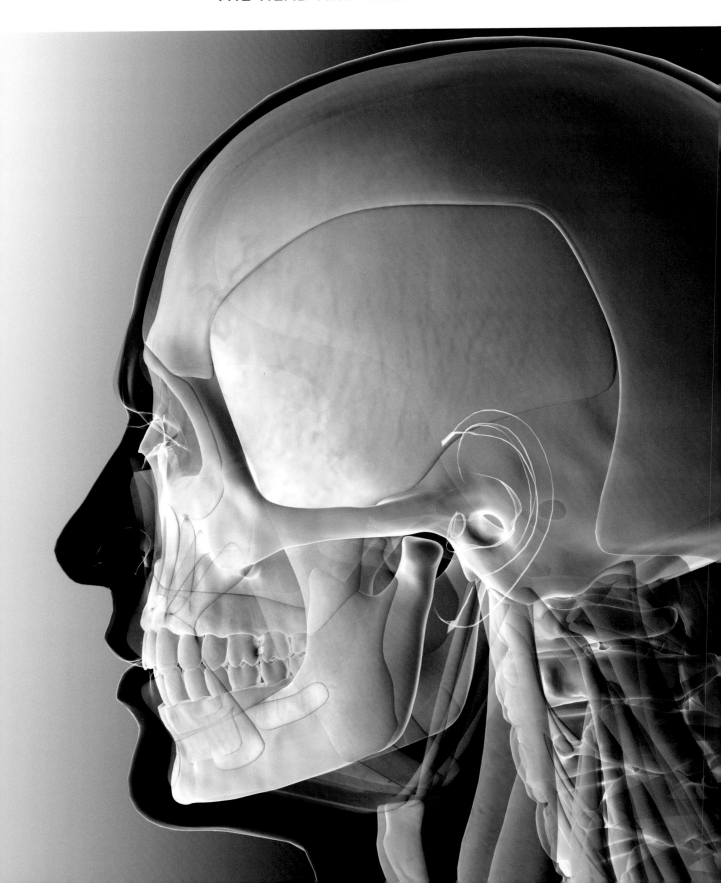

bones to heal or change. The skeleton of a fetus is made of cartilage that gradually changes to bone in a process called ossification. From birth to adolescence bones continually grow and develop. Although adult bones can no longer grow, they are able to renew, remodel, or strengthen—thanks to the periosteum—in response to stress. The cells that remodel bones are called osteoclasts (which break cells down) and osteoblasts (which build cells up). Osteoblasts develop growing bones in children and adolescents.

The head houses the brain, an organ that is the body's control system. The brain, a jellylike substance that weighs about 3 pounds (1.4 kilograms) in an adult, is protected by the skull and its cranial bones. The head also houses the sensory organs for seeing, hearing, smelling, and tasting. These organs are the eyes, the ears, the nose, and the tongue. Their proximity to the brain ensures rapid processing of the complex information they gather from the environment.

The brain itself is divided into three parts: the brain stem, which is an extension of the spinal cord; the forebrain, which consists mainly of the cerebrum; and the cerebellum. The forebrain and cerebrum are divided into two hemispheres that are linked by a thick band of nerve fibers known as the corpus callosum. The wiring system of the brain is "crossed," that is, the right cerebral hemisphere

ll and spinal column work together to connect the head to the rest of y and to keep communication flowing to and from the brain.

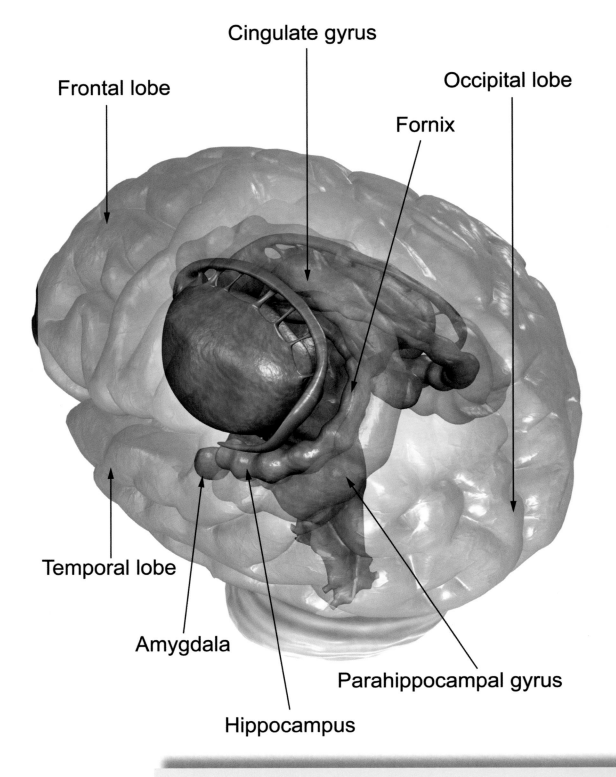

Cingulate gyrus

Frontal lobe

Occipital lobe

Fornix

Temporal lobe

Amygdala

Parahippocampal gyrus

Hippocampus

The brain is a complex organ with different areas responsible for different functions.

controls the left side of the body and vice versa. Three layers of connective tissue membranes, known as meninges, along with

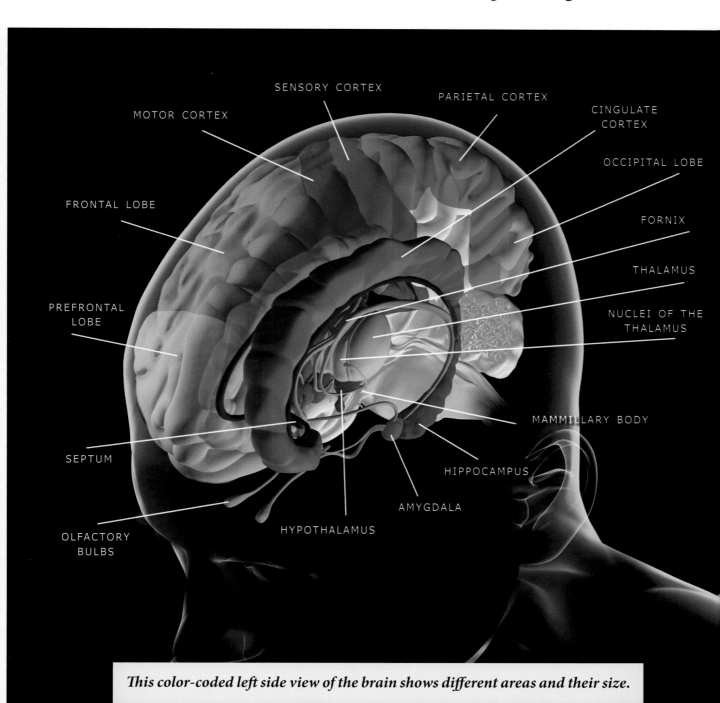

SENSORY CORTEX

PARIETAL CORTEX

CINGULATE CORTEX

MOTOR CORTEX

OCCIPITAL LOBE

FRONTAL LOBE

FORNIX

THALAMUS

PREFRONTAL LOBE

NUCLEI OF THE THALAMUS

MAMMILLARY BODY

SEPTUM

HIPPOCAMPUS

AMYGDALA

HYPOTHALAMUS

OLFACTORY BULBS

This color-coded left side view of the brain shows different areas and their size.

THE HARD-WORKING BRAIN

The brain requires large amounts of stored energy for thinking. This is why people may feel as tired after studying hard as they would after playing a strenuous sport or a physical workout. One of the hardest-working parts of the body, the brain doesn't even stop working immediately after a person dies. It continues to send out electrical signals for about thirty-seven hours after death.

spaces filled with cerebrospinal fluid, surround and cushion the brain from shocks or injury when the head hits something.

THE HUMAN SKULL

The human skull is the bony section of the head. It encases and protects the brain and provides attachments for the muscles of the head and neck. The skull consists of two sets of bones: cranial bones and facial bones. They protect and support the organs that are responsible for the five basic senses: sight, hearing, smell, taste, and touch. The front of the skull also features two orbits, cuplike sockets or hollow places that hold the eyes.

In the bones of the forehead and cheeks are air-filled spaces called sinuses. The sinuses in the bones that surround the nasal cavity, the hole in the middle of the face, are called the paranasal sinuses. They are cavities in the bones of the face that are lined

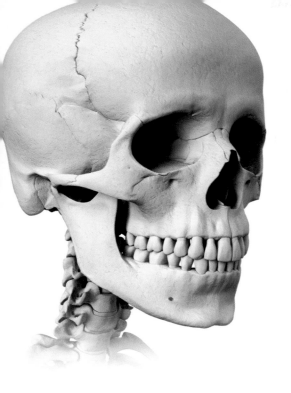

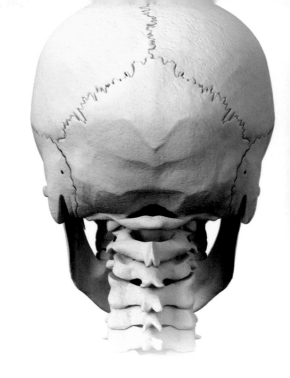

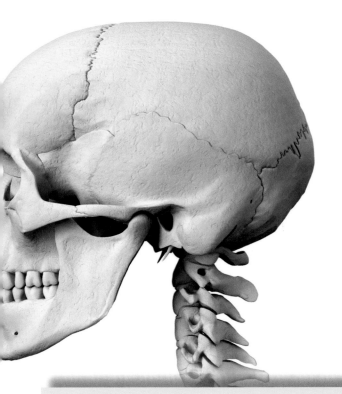

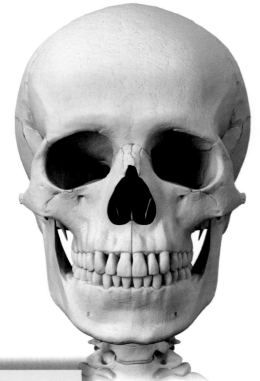

The purpose of the human skull is to protect the brain and other organs of the head and neck, as well as to facilitate movement.

with mucous membranes. The mucus produced in the sinuses drains into the nasal cavity to moisturize and warm the air as it flows into the respiratory tract. When drainage from the paranasal sinuses is blocked, such as during a cold, the sinuses often become affected and cause headaches or other discomforts.

Most of the nose is composed of soft, springy cartilage, but the base of the nose is bone. The maxilla is the bone of the upper jaw. The mandible is the bone of the lower jaw. The mandible is one of the few bones in the head that can move. The muscles that move it are anchored to the cheekbones and the sides of the skull.

The part of the skull that encloses the brain is the cranium, or "brainbox." Its eight bones are thin and flat and interlock at their joints so they cannot move. The frontal bone forms the forehead and upper part of the eye sockets. Two parietal bones form the sides and upper portion of the cranium.

Under the parietal bones are two temporal bones, one on each side of the skull. They join the parietal bone along the squamosal suture. Temporal bones form parts of the sides and base of the cranium. The occipital bone forms the back of the cranium. Temporal bones house the internal structures of the ear. They have depressions, the mandibular fossae, where the mandible, the bone of the lower jaw, attaches to the temporal bones.

Teeth are hard structures in the upper and lower jaw that aid in chewing food and in the process of speaking clearly, as well as giving shape to the face. The hardest substance in the human body, even harder than bone, is enamel, one of the four kinds of tissue that make up a tooth. Enamel covers the crown

Skull Anatomy

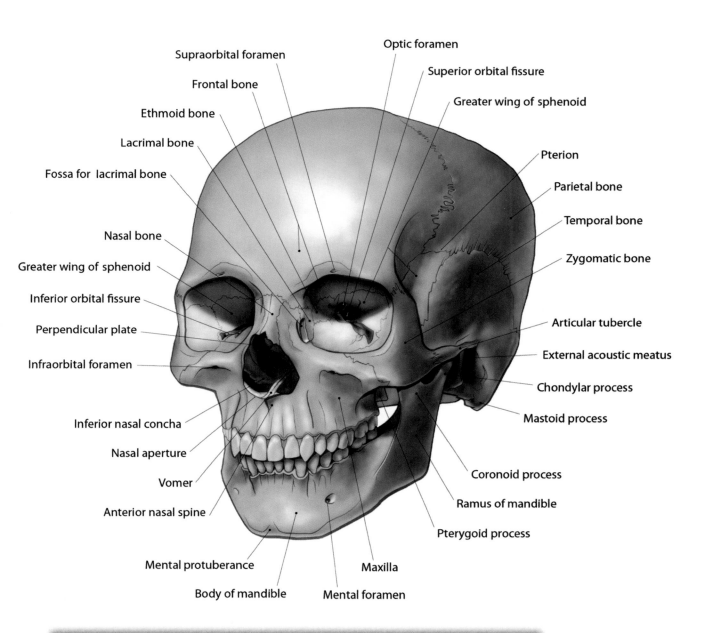

Supraorbital foramen

Frontal bone

Ethmoid bone

Lacrimal bone

Fossa for lacrimal bone

Nasal bone

Greater wing of sphenoid

Inferior orbital fissure

Perpendicular plate

Infraorbital foramen

Inferior nasal concha

Nasal aperture

Vomer

Anterior nasal spine

Mental protuberance

Body of mandible

Optic foramen

Superior orbital fissure

Greater wing of sphenoid

Pterion

Parietal bone

Temporal bone

Zygomatic bone

Articular tubercle

External acoustic meatus

Chondylar process

Mastoid process

Coronoid process

Ramus of mandible

Pterygoid process

Maxilla

Mental foramen

The human skull consists of twenty-two bones and can be broken into many different areas as shown here.

of the tooth, the area above the gum line. A bony material, the cementum, covers the root, which fits into the jaw socket and is joined to it with membranes. At the heart of each tooth is living pulp, which contains nerves, connective tissues, blood vessels, and lymphatic tissue. When we get a toothache, it is the nerve inside the pulp that hurts.

There are fourteen bones in the face. As mentioned, some facial bones contain hollow, air-filled spaces known as sinuses. The main function of the sinuses is to lighten the skull and to provide sound quality for the voice.

Bones not considered part of the skull but associated with it include the bones of the middle ear and the hyoid bone. Three auditory bones inside each middle ear cavity transmit vibrations from the eardrum to receptors in the inner ear. Those bones are the incus, the stapes, and the malleus. The horseshoe-shaped hyoid bone is suspended by ligaments from the lower portions of the temporal bones. It lies in the neck just above the larynx (voice box). It plays an important part in swallowing and supporting the tongue and larynx.

A skull fracture is a break in one or more of the skull bones caused by a blow to the head. Since the skull is very strong, most fractures close by themselves and cause no complications. Young people at play without a helmet may suffer skull fractures by falling from a bicycle or skateboard or by being hit by a bat or a ball. Anyone suffering a violent blow to the head, especially if it causes unconsciousness, should see a doctor since skull fractures can result in brain injury.

The upper spinal cord and cervical vertebrae both support the head and carry signals from the brain to other parts of the body.

THE NECK

The neck supports the head, enables it to move, and provides a link between the head and the trunk of the body. Supporting the neck are seven cervical vertebrae; the top two allow the head to move from side to side and up and down.

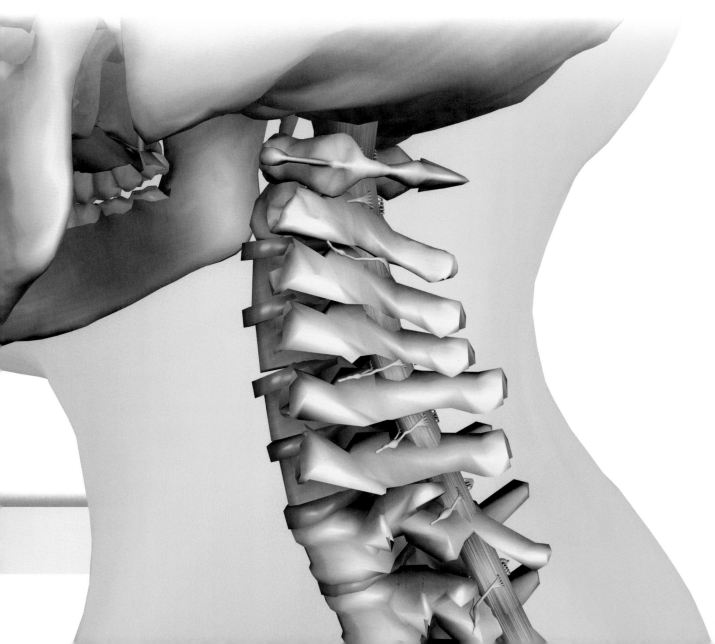

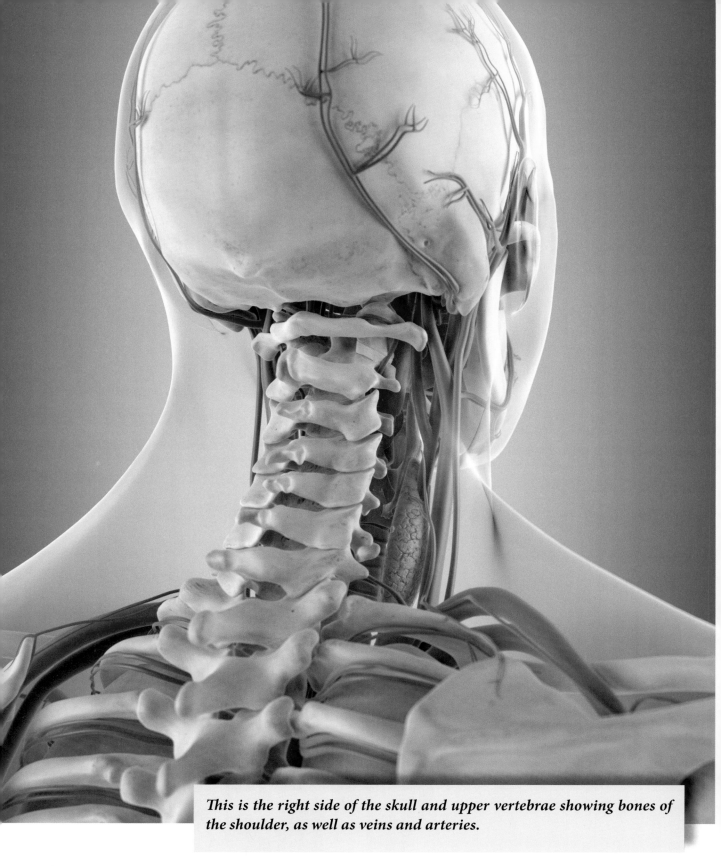

This is the right side of the skull and upper vertebrae showing bones of the shoulder, as well as veins and arteries.

The neck contains the larynx, or "voice box," composed mostly of muscles and cartilage that are bound together by elastic tissues. The thyroid cartilage was named for the thyroid gland that covers its lower part. This cartilage is the shieldlike structure that protrudes in the front of the neck and is called the Adam's apple. It is usually more prominent in males than in females because of the effect of male sex hormones on the development of the larynx.

The trachea, or "windpipe," begins immediately below the larynx and runs down the center of the front part of the neck, ending behind the upper part of the sternum. It then divides to form two branches that enter the lung cavities. The trachea is made up of fibrous and elastic tissues and smooth muscle with about twenty rings of cartilage that help keep the trachea open during extreme neck movements.

The spine is the body's "backbone," a strong, curved, rod-like series of thirty-three bones called vertebrae that support the main parts of the body in an upright position. Supporting the skull on the spine is the first vertebra, or atlas, at a joint that allows for nodding and other head and neck movements. It is called the atlas because in Greek mythology, after leading the Titans in an unsuccessful war against the Olympians, the god Atlas was condemned to hold the sky on his shoulders for all eternity. This was the mythological explanation for what holds up the sky.

The first vertebra has a ringlike socket into which fits a peg from the second vertebra, called the axis. Two rounded bumps under the skull fit into the hollows on the atlas and

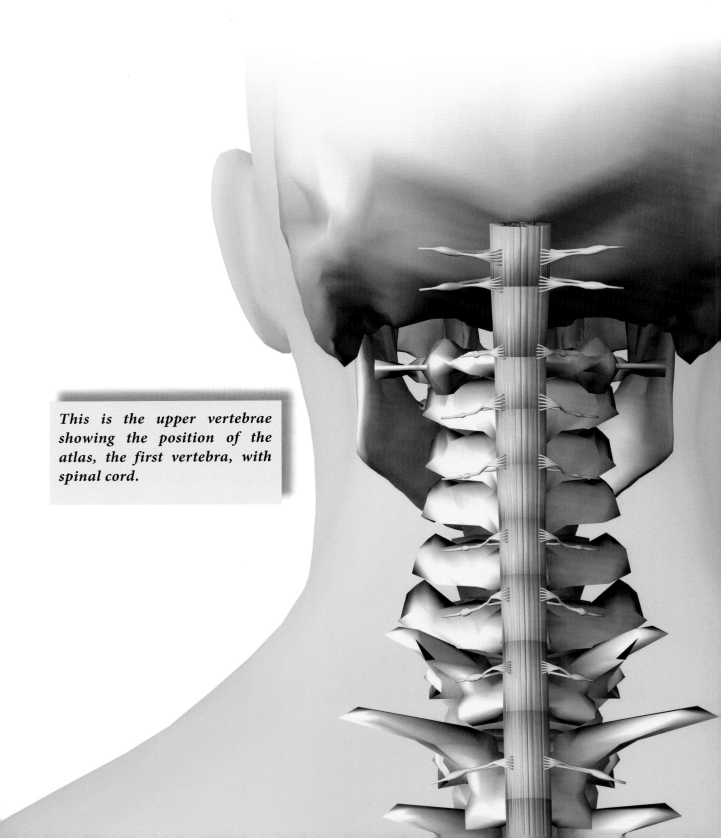

This is the upper vertebrae showing the position of the atlas, the first vertebra, with spinal cord.

allow nodding movement. The muscles of the posterior of the neck, such as the splenius capitis and semispinalis capitis, assisted by the trapezius, support the head by pulling it back to keep it from falling forward.

The spinal cord is the brain's main link with the rest of the body. It is a cable about 17 inches (43 centimeters) long that descends from the brain stem to the lumbar part of the back. Through thirty-one pairs of spinal nerves, the spinal cord is connected to the rest of the body and relays information from the sensory nerves to the brain and from the brain to the motor nerves. The brain and nerves make up the body's nervous system.

Injuries to the head and neck can cause paralysis. In 1995, Christopher Reeve, the athletic young actor who played Superman in the 1970s and 1980s movies, fell from his horse and landed on his head. The first and second cervical vertebrae, those closest to the skull, had been shattered. Severe damage to his spinal cord left Reeve a quadriplegic, unable to move his arms and legs. Scientists and doctors are experimenting with ways to repair damaged or severed spinal cords and restore two-way communication up and down the spine.

CHAPTER TWO

MUSCLES OF THE HEAD AND NECK

The muscles are fleshy tissues connected to the bones that control articulation, including flexion and extension (nodding) and rotation (shaking the head). Muscles contract (shorten) or relax (lengthen) in response to nerve impulses. The muscles of the head and neck include neck and throat muscles that allow the head to nod, shake, and swivel and also control the movements of the lower lip. Jaw and mouth muscles help us to chew and swallow. Eye muscles open and close the eyelids and govern some facial expressions. Eye movement itself is controlled by six muscles inside of the eyeball that allow the eye to move in any direction. The cranial muscles cover most of the skull and allow our eyebrows to move.

Muscles are not able to stretch, but they contract and relax under stimulus from nerve cells attached to them. Each muscle is made of hundreds to thousands of

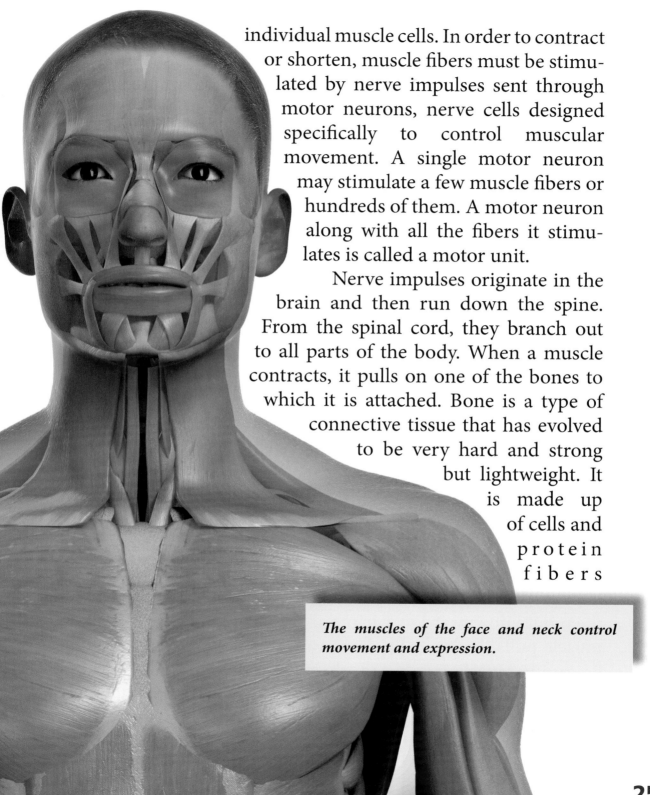

individual muscle cells. In order to contract or shorten, muscle fibers must be stimulated by nerve impulses sent through motor neurons, nerve cells designed specifically to control muscular movement. A single motor neuron may stimulate a few muscle fibers or hundreds of them. A motor neuron along with all the fibers it stimulates is called a motor unit.

Nerve impulses originate in the brain and then run down the spine. From the spinal cord, they branch out to all parts of the body. When a muscle contracts, it pulls on one of the bones to which it is attached. Bone is a type of connective tissue that has evolved to be very hard and strong but lightweight. It is made up of cells and protein fibers

The muscles of the face and neck control movement and expression.

interwoven into a hard, calcified matrix that is porous—that is, full of small cavities, empty spaces that reduce its weight. Many facial muscles are not attached to bones but to each other or to the skin. Which muscle contracts when, and with what force, is controlled and coordinated by the brain, in the case of voluntary movements.

When we smile, frown, or open our mouth to speak or shout, we use one or more of over thirty small facial muscles. Most facial muscles are in pairs, one on each side of the face. The muscles pull on the skin of the face, changing its shape. Larger muscles move the head and keep it upright. They also close the lower jaw when we eat or speak.

FACIAL MUSCLES

Seven muscles in the front of the face do different things. The frontalis muscle pulls the scalp forward to wrinkle the forehead and raise the eyebrows. The orbicularis oculi muscle surrounds the eye sockets and closes the eyes. The levator labii superioris muscle raises the upper lip and flares the nostrils when we demonstrate disgust for something.

The orbicularis oris muscle surrounds the mouth and closes the lips. The depressor anguli oris muscle draws the corners of the mouth downward in a grimace. The depressor labii inferioris muscle pulls the lower lip downward in a pout. The semispinalis capitis muscle is a broad, sheetlike muscle that extends up from the vertebrae in the neck and thorax to the occipital bone.

Anterior Head and Neck Facial Muscles

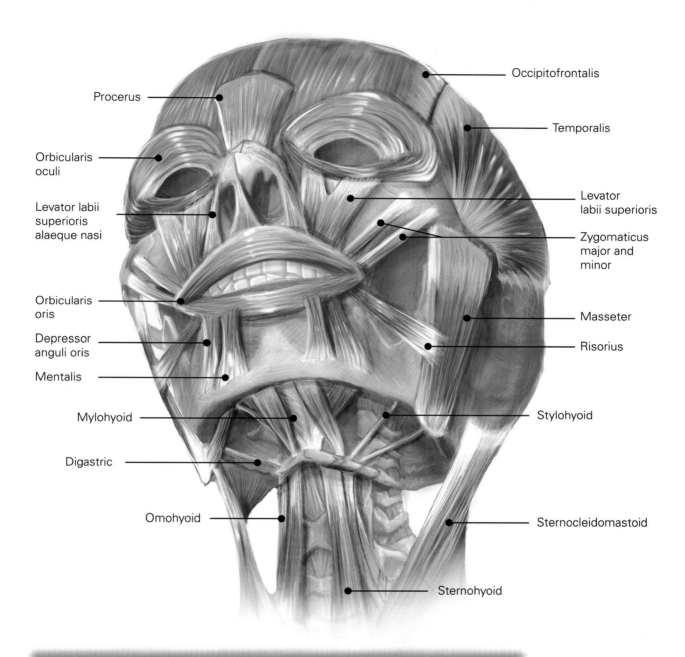

Procerus

Orbicularis oculi

Levator labii superioris alaeque nasi

Orbicularis oris

Depressor anguli oris

Mentalis

Mylohyoid

Digastric

Omohyoid

Occipitofrontalis

Temporalis

Levator labii superioris

Zygomaticus major and minor

Masseter

Risorius

Stylohyoid

Sternocleidomastoid

Sternohyoid

The head, neck, and facial muscles control our ability to breathe, eat, speak, and express ourselves nonverbally.

It extends the head, bends it to one side, and rotates it.

The platysma muscle in the side of the chin and neck draws the lower lip and corners of the mouth sideways and down, partially opening the mouth, as in an expression of doubt, rejection, surprise, or fright. It is a broad sheet of muscle arising from the pectoral (chest) and deltoid (shoulder) muscles and rises over the clavicle (collarbone), proceeding upward in a slanting manner along the sides of the neck.

All skeletal muscles, including those in the head and neck, have the same basic features. The center of the muscle, called the belly, is attached to bones or other structures at each end. But the shape, power, and mobility of individual muscles depend on how their fascicles are arranged. Fascicles are bundles of muscle fibers. Their number

The facial muscles relative to the skull.

and orientation determine how powerful muscles are and in what direction they will contract or relax.

There are three types of muscles in the head and neck: parallel muscles, pennate muscles, and circular muscles. Parallel muscles have fascicles arranged parallel to the long axis of the muscle. They can be fusiform, with a fleshy belly, such as the biceps femoris in the upper arm. Or they can be straplike, such as the sartorius in the thigh.

Pennate muscles have fascicles arranged obliquely (at an angle, neither parallel nor perpendicular) to a tendon running along the center of the muscle. These muscles can be unipennate, with fascicles attached to one side of the tendon, such as the extensor digitorum longus in the lower leg. Bipennate muscles have fascicles attached like a feather to both sides of the central tendon, such as the rectus femoris in the thigh. Multipennate muscles are those with many bipennate units, such as the deltoid muscle in the shoulder.

Circular muscles are those with concentric (circular or spherical) rows of fascicles. They form a sphincter muscle that controls the closing of external body openings, such as the orbicularis oculi muscle around the eyes. The sphincter muscle contracts when the eyelids close. Six pairs of muscles control the almost constant movements of the eyeballs.

A sphincter muscle also forms a large part of the lips. Seven pairs of muscles control movements of the mouth that turn the corners of the mouth up or down, or in and out. Movements of the jaw are controlled by four different pairs of muscles. Of these, the temporalis and masseter muscles are very powerful sets of

MUSCLE FACTS

It takes seventeen muscles to make a smile but forty-three muscles to make a frown. The smallest muscle in the human body is the stapedius muscle in the ear, just 0.05 inch (0.13 cm) long. It activates the stirrup, the small bone that sends vibrations from the eardrum to the inner ear. The fastest-reacting muscle in the human body is the orbicularis oculi, which encircles the eye and closes the eyelid. It contracts in less than 0.01 second.

muscles that raise the lower jaw and close the mouth during eating and chewing.

THE MUSCLES OF THE SIDE AND BACK OF THE HEAD

Other muscles at the side and back of the head and neck control additional facial expressions and support and move the head and neck.

The risorius muscle pulls the corners of the lips laterally (sideways) when we smile. The zygomaticus muscle pulls the corners of the mouth up and out when we smile or laugh. The corrugator supercilii muscle wrinkles the brow when we frown. The buccinator (cheek muscle) pushes the cheeks inward when

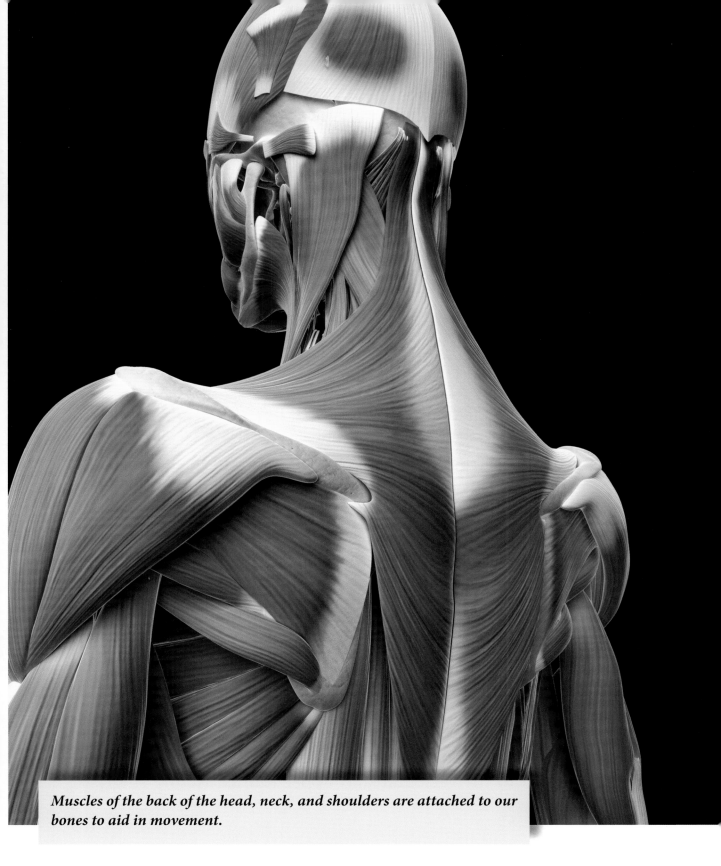

Muscles of the back of the head, neck, and shoulders are attached to our bones to aid in movement.

we suck on something and also forces food inward between the teeth during chewing.

As mentioned, two powerful muscles, the temporalis and masseter, raise the lower jaw to close the mouth. The occipitalis muscle, at the back of the skull, is linked to the frontalis by a flat tendon, the galea aponeurotica, the muscle that covers the upper part of the skull. Attached to the frontal and occipital bellies (muscles on the brow at the front and on the upper back of the head), it moves the scalp freely over the underlying skull bone. The occipital and frontal bellies work together with this muscle to draw back the scalp, raise the eyebrows, and wrinkle the forehead in an expression of surprise.

The sternocleidomastoid muscles flex the head, pulling it toward the chest. They are long muscles on the sides of the neck that extend up from the thorax to the base of the skull behind the ear. When this muscle on one side of the head contracts, the face turns to the opposite side. When both muscles contract, the head bends toward the chest.

While a sternocleidomastoid muscle acting individually rotates the head to one side, the trapezius muscle has an opposing action, pulling the head and shoulders backward. It is a flat, triangular muscle that covers the back of the neck, shoulders, and thorax.

Lying deep in the neck on either side are the cervical plexus muscles. They are connected to the front branches of the first four cervical nerves. In the back of the neck is the splenius capitis muscle. It is a broad, straplike muscle that connects the base of the skull to the vertebrae and upper thorax. Acting singly, a

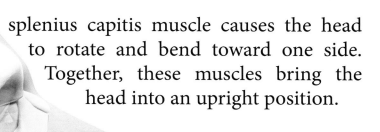

splenius capitis muscle causes the head to rotate and bend toward one side. Together, these muscles bring the head into an upright position.

HOW MUSCLES MOVE

Almost all movements of the body result from muscle contraction. Even when at rest or asleep, muscle fibers contract to maintain muscle tone and good health. Muscle activity generates heat, which is vital in maintaining normal body temperature.

An individual skeletal muscle fiber is from 1/16 of an inch to

The bones of the head and neck showing movement.

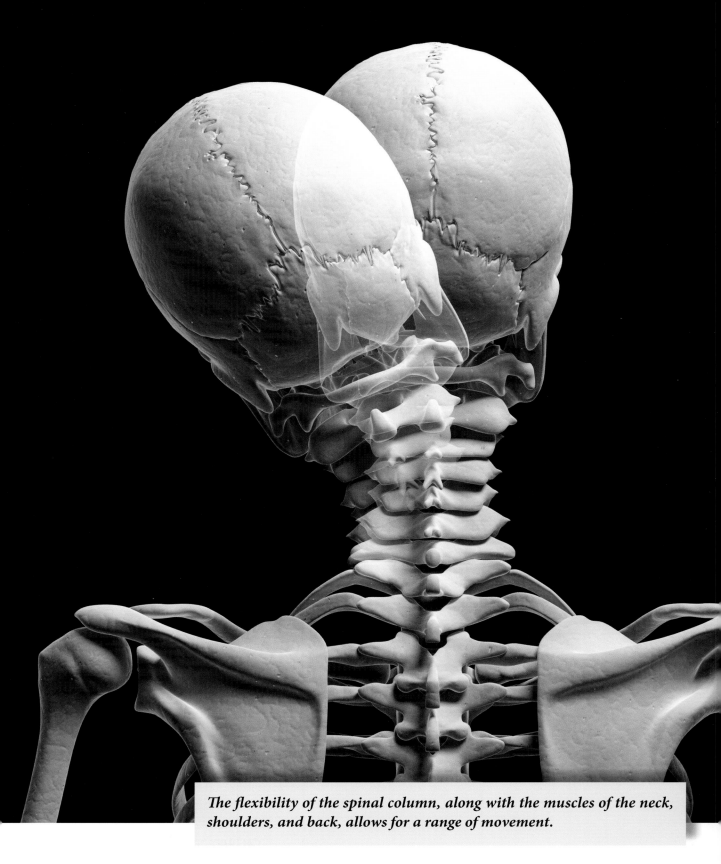

The flexibility of the spinal column, along with the muscles of the neck, shoulders, and back, allows for a range of movement.

12 inches (1 millimeter to 30 centimeters) long. As we have said, in order to contract or shorten, muscle fibers have to be stimulated by nerve impulses sent through motor neurons or nerves. When a motor neuron reaches a muscle fiber, it fits into a hollow on the surface of the muscle fiber. When a nerve impulse reaches the end of the motor neuron, a neurotransmitter, a chemical called acetylcholine, is released. This chemical crosses the small gap between the motor neuron and the muscle fiber and attaches to receptors on the membrane of the muscle fiber. This sets off an electrical charge that travels rapidly from one end of the muscle fiber to the other, causing it to contract.

CHAPTER THREE

SENSORY ORGANS

The sensory organs are an extension of the central nervous system. Their only function is to send information to the brain. Sense organs are stimulated constantly and send a steady stream of information about changes in the environment that a person gets via touch, smell, vision, hearing, or taste.

TASTE

Both taste and smell are chemical senses, stimulated by chemical molecules. Tastes are detected by special structures called gustatory cayculi, or "taste buds." Humans have about ten thousand taste buds, mainly on the tongue, but a few at the back of the throat and on the palate, the top of the mouth.

There are four types of taste buds. They are sensitive to sweet, salty, sour, and bitter substances. Each taste receptor is most highly concentrated in certain regions of the tongue's surface. Sweet receptors are mostly on the tip of the tongue, sour receptors are mainly along the sides of the tongue, salt receptors are most common in the tip (apex) and upper front portion of the tongue,

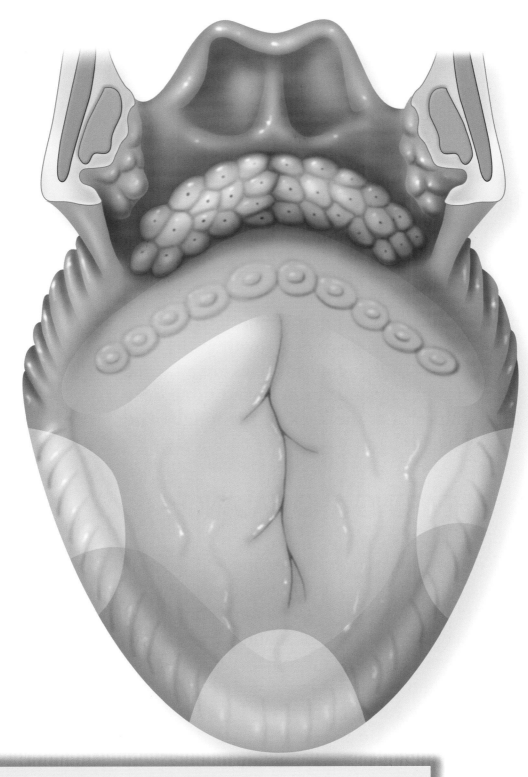

This is a map of taste regions of the tongue. Bitter is green, sour is pink, sweet is purple, and salt is yellow.

and bitter receptors are located toward the back of the tongue.

The tongue's many muscles allow for sucking, swallowing, and making sounds to produce speech and song. Most of the tongue consists of closely interlaced muscles arranged in pairs so that the left and right sides of the tongue have independent sets of muscles.

The tongue is anchored to the floor of the mouth and at the rear of the mouth from muscles attached to a spiky outgrowth at the base of the skull. The tongue's muscles are attached to the lower jaw and to the hyoid bone deep in the muscles at the back of the tongue and above the larynx.

HEARING AND BALANCE

The ear, an organ for both hearing and balance, consists of three parts: the outer ear, the middle ear, and the inner ear. The outer and middle ear mainly collect and transmit sound. The inner ear analyzes sound waves and contains an apparatus that maintains the body's balance.

The outer ear is the part that is visible and is made of folds of skin and cartilage. It leads into the ear canal, which is closed at the inner end by the

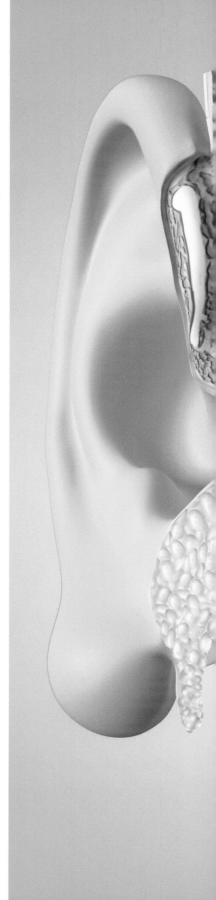

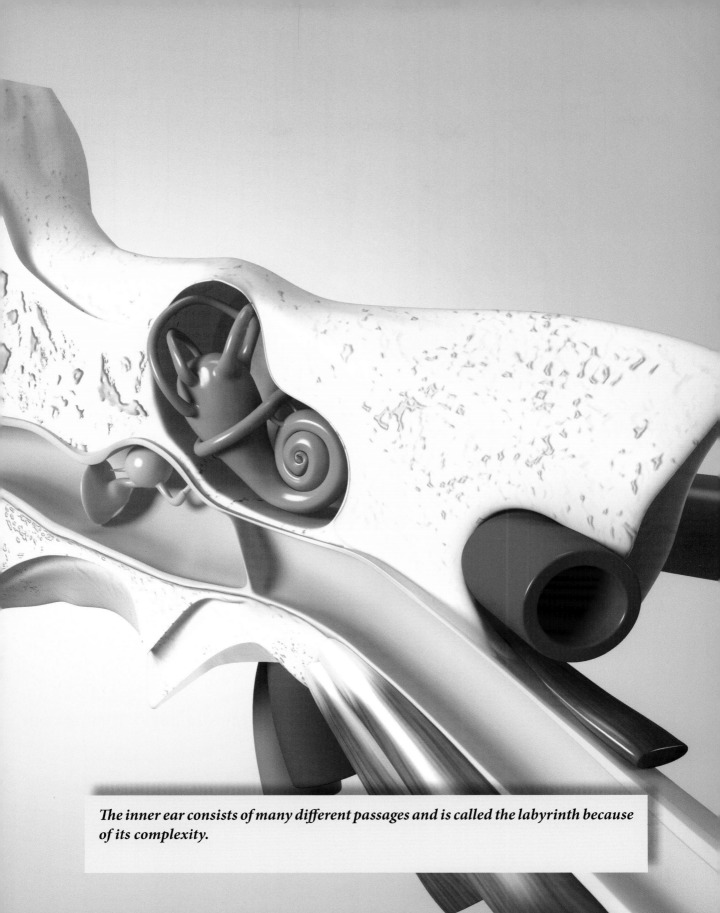

The inner ear consists of many different passages and is called the labyrinth because of its complexity.

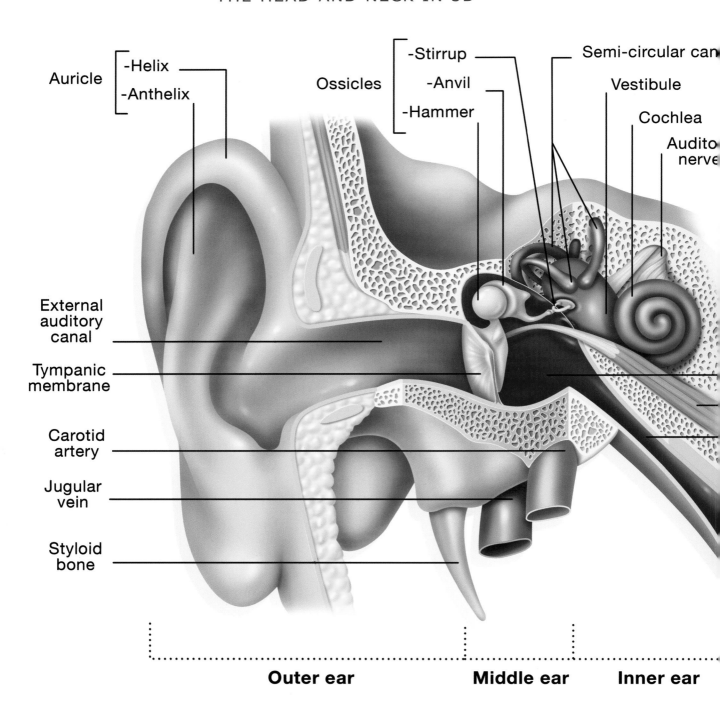

Auricle
- -Helix
- -Anthelix

Ossicles
- -Stirrup
- -Anvil
- -Hammer

Semi-circular can

Vestibule

Cochlea

Audito
nerve

External auditory canal

Tympanic membrane

Carotid artery

Jugular vein

Styloid bone

Outer ear

Middle ear

Inner ear

The outer and inner ear are made up of several parts.

eardrum. Sound enters the ear through the ear canal and strikes the tympanic membrane. Resulting vibrations affect three bones in the middle ear—the malleus (also called the "hammer" in the diagram above), incus (or "anvil"), and stapes (also called the "stirrup")—that in turn pass the vibrations into the cochlea to the organ of corti. Impulses from this organ travel to the brain to be interpreted as sound.

The middle ear or tympanic cavity is a small, irregular, laterally compressed space within the temporal bone. It is filled with air sent from the nasal part of the pharynx through the auditory tube. It contains a chain of three tiny, movable bones called ossicles. They connect to the middle ear's medial wall and serve to convey the vibrations sent to the tympanic membrane across the cavity to the internal ear. Ossicles are the smallest bones in the human body.

The inner ear is a very delicate series of structures deep within the bones of the skull. It consists of a maze of winding passages called the labyrinth. The front is a tube that looks like a snail's shell and is concerned with hearing. The rear part is concerned with balance.

Impaired hearing and deafness may occur because of nerve deafness in the ears. Cilia on the sense receptors within the cochlea may have worn away, which can happen with age. Nerve deafness also may occur by listening frequently to loud sounds such as music amplified above 130 decibels.

Tympanic cavity

Hammer muscle

Eustachian tube

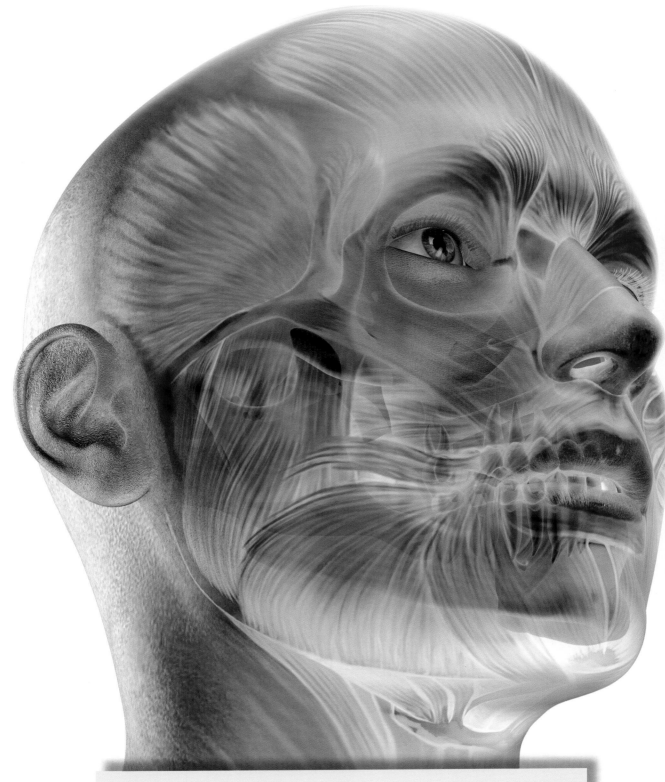

The bones, muscles, and skin cover the sensory organs of the head and neck.

MAKING SENSE WITH SENSES

The human nose can distinguish between fifty thousand different smells. Every three to four hours our nostrils switch duty; one keeps smelling and breathing while the other rests. Earwax comes from a combination of body oil and sweat. If you stand on your head while swallowing, the food would not go down but up because muscles in the esophagus would still pull the food into the stomach.

SMELL

The nose is both the sensory organ that identifies smells and the main airway for the respiratory system. Inside the nose is the olfactory epithelium, a small patch of nerve cells with hairy projections. These are covered with receptors sensitive to the molecules of various substances in the air. There are about ten million receptors in the nose, of at least twenty different types. When the receptors detect an odor, they send nerve signals along the olfactory nerve to the smell center in the brain. There the signal pattern is analyzed and the smell is identified.

The peripheral olfactory organ, or the organ of smell, consists of two parts: an outer part, the external nose that projects from the center of the face and an inner part, the nasal cavity that is divided by a septum into right and left nasal chambers.

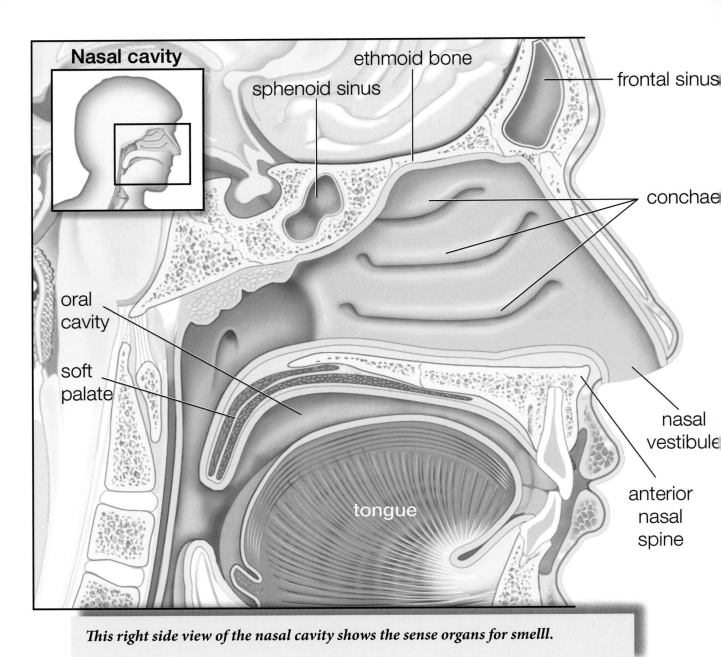

Nasal cavity

ethmoid bone

sphenoid sinus

frontal sinus

conchae

oral cavity

soft palate

nasal vestibule

anterior nasal spine

tongue

This right side view of the nasal cavity shows the sense organs for smelll.

The external nose is composed of bones and cartilage. Shaped like a pyramid, its upper angle or root connects directly with the forehead. Its free angle is termed the apex. Its base is perforated by two elliptical orifices, the rares, separated from each other by the columna.

The internal nose contains two nasal cavities, narrow canals with lateral walls separated from one another by a wall composed of bone and cartilage. Special cells in the narrow upper parts of the nasal cavities act as odor receptors. Nerves lead from these cells to the brain, where impulses generated by the odor receptors are interpreted as smell.

As air passes through the nasal cavity with each inhalation, both gaseous and solid particles travel with it, causing stimulation of the olfactory bulbs. Impulses from these go to the brain where the sensation of smell occurs rapidly. During exhaling, the air passes below the olfactory bulbs.

The adenoids, two glands at the back of the nose above the tonsils, are made up of lymph node tissue that contains white cells to defend the body in fighting infection. The adenoids tend to enlarge during early childhood, before the age of five or six, but usually disappear by puberty.

ORGANS OF THE NECK AND THROAT

Glossopharyngeal nerves, the ninth pair of cranial nerves, are associated with the tongue and pharynx. They are primarily sensory nerves. The fibers carry impulses to the brain from the lining of the pharynx, tonsils, and rear portion of the tongue. Fibers in the

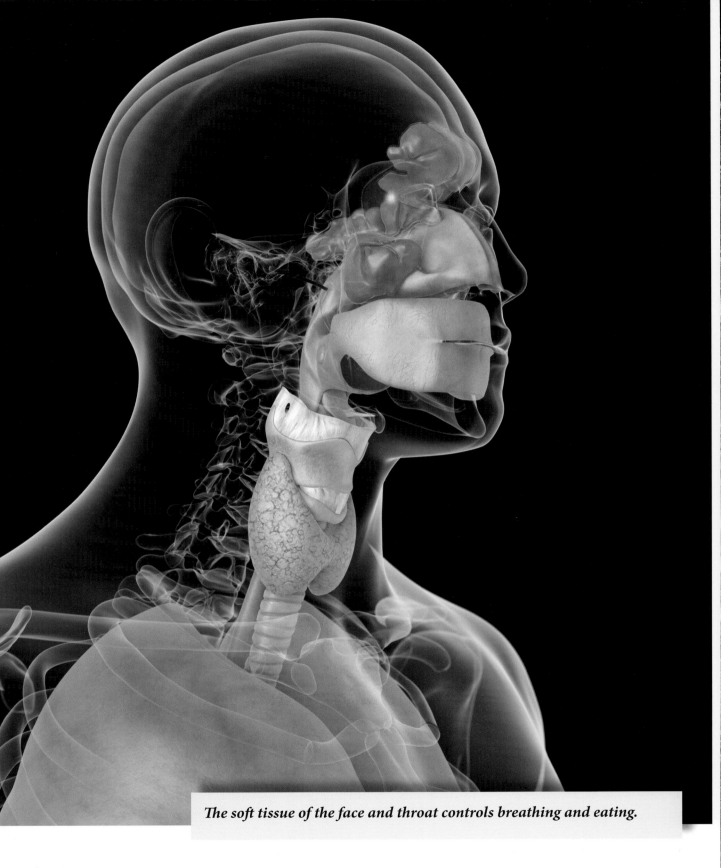

The soft tissue of the face and throat controls breathing and eating.

motor components aid in swallowing.

As food enters the back of the pharynx, a flap (the epiglottis) keeps food from entering the trachea and lungs. The food passes into the esophagus and down into the stomach. During swallowing, the soft palate and uvula are drawn upward, closing the portion of the pharynx opening to the nose, preventing food and fluid from entering the nasal cavity.

The esophagus is a muscular tube that carries food and liquids from the throat to the stomach for digestion after it has been chewed and

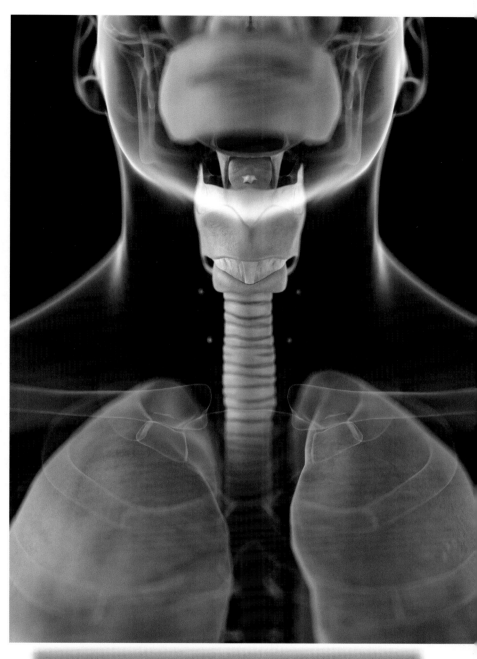

A front view of the larynx.

chemically softened in the mouth. Food is forced downward to the stomach by powerful waves of muscle contractions passing through the walls of the esophagus. If the food tastes really awful or is poisonous, it may travel back by the action of the same muscles and be thrown out through the mouth, which is called vomiting.

The tonsils are a pair of oval-shaped organs in the back of the throat. They are part of the lymphatic system, which is important to the body's defense against infection. Like the adenoids at the base of the tongue, the tonsils protect against upper respiratory tract infections. They enlarge from birth to about seven years of age, then shrink.

SIGHT

While the eyes, the sensory organs for vision, are at the front of the head, the actual site where visual images are interpreted and created is at the back and sides of the brain. Light rays enter the eye through the cornea, an opening at the front of the eye. The light rays fall upon the retina, a layer of small, thin, light-sensitive cells at the back of the eyeball. The eye generates patterns of nerve signals and sends them to the brain.

Nerve impulses from rods and cones, cells that respond to light and color, in the retinas of the eyes travel along the optic nerves, the second pair of the cranial nerves, to the optic chiasma, where they cross over each other. Rods are responsible for vision in dim light and create a black-and-white image. Cones create fine detail and are sensitive to color. Impulses from both eyes pass through the optic

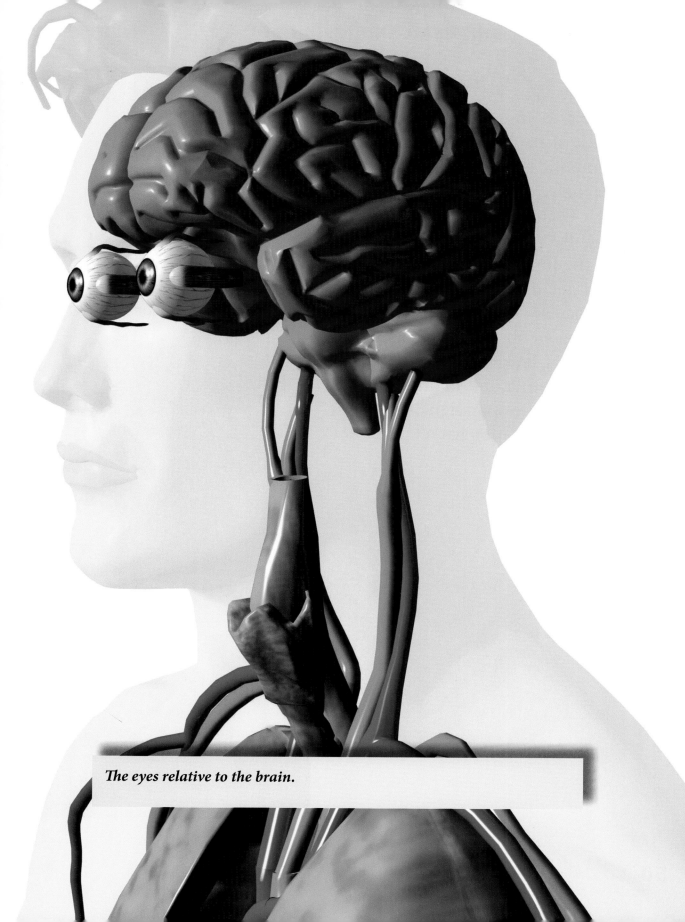

The eyes relative to the brain.

tracts to the striate cortex at the back of the brain. They end in the temporal lobe area, where right and left halves of the visual field merge.

Each eye sees objects from a slightly different angle. The fusion of the images from both eyes gives a three-dimensional effect called binocular or stereoscopic vision. Seeing an object and recognizing it involves image processing by cells in the retina and brain. The brain analyzes the optic signals and identifies information from them.

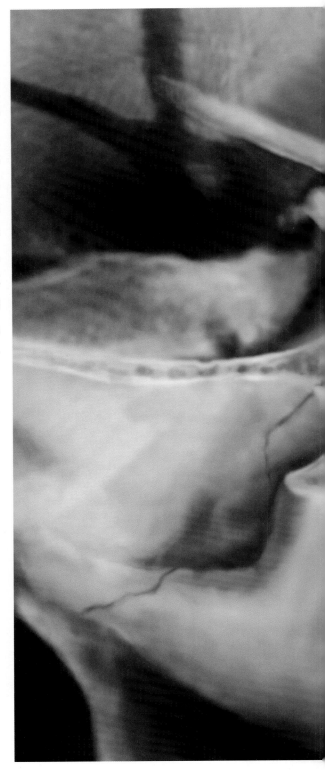

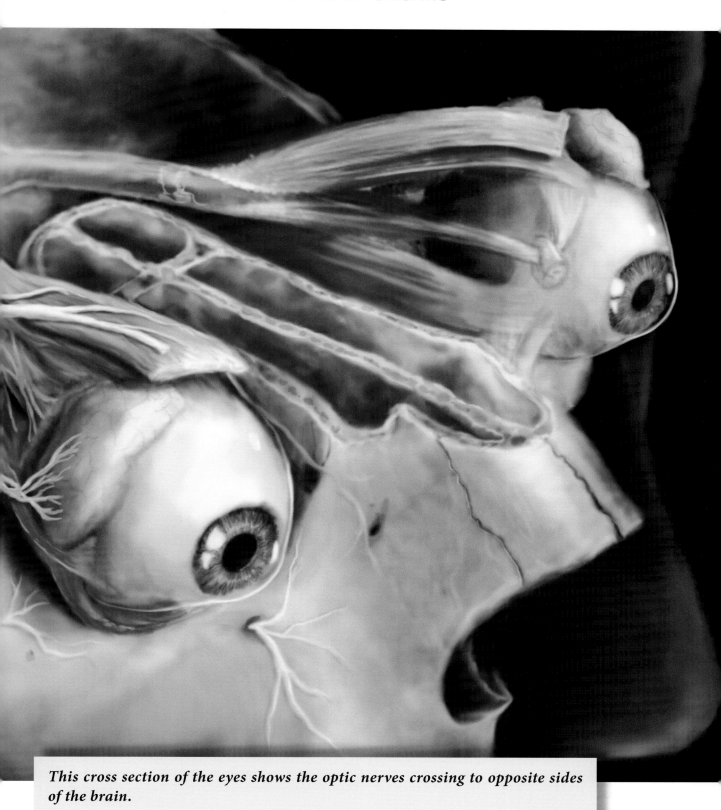

This cross section of the eyes shows the optic nerves crossing to opposite sides of the brain.

CONCLUSION

In this book we have focused on the bones, the muscles, and the organs of the head and neck. This part of the anatomy is usually broken down into the various systems which operate in the head and neck. These include the musculoskeletal system (the bones and muscles covered in chapters one and two), the circulatory system (through which blood circulates via veins and arteries), the nervous system (including the brain, spinal cords and nerves), and the respiratory system (the nose and mouth through which air is filtered to the lungs). By addressing these areas, we have taken a look beneath the skin to the inside of the body. However, it is important to note that without the skin, these systems would not be able to function.

GLOSSARY

ANATOMY The structure or form of a living thing.

ARTERIES Tubes that carry blood from the heart to different parts of the body.

BONE A strong part of the body's skeletal structure composed mainly of calcium compounds.

BRAIN An organ in the skull that controls and coordinates the body's mental and physical actions.

CARTILAGE A tough, rubbery connective tissue that lines the ends of bones where they meet a joint.

CIRCULATORY SYSTEM A system that is made up of blood, blood vessels, and the heart.

CONE A receptor cell in the retina of the eye that detects color and provides visual sharpness.

FIBERS Thin, threadlike structures in muscles that facilitate movement by shortening and lengthening.

INNER EAR The part of the ear where balance is maintained and sound is transmitted.

JOINT A connection between two or more bones.

LARYNX The organ containing the vocal cords, also called the voice box.

LIGAMENTS Fibrous tissues that hold bones together and connect joints.

MANDIBLE The lower jaw.

MIDDLE EAR The air-filled cavity of the ear where sound is amplified.

MUSCULOSKELETAL SYSTEM A system of muscles and bones that work together to facilitate movement.

NERVOUS SYSTEM A system of nerves in the body that sends messages to the brain and controls the sensation of touch and movement.

ORGAN A major structural part of the body, usually a collection of tissues, that carries out a specific function.

OSSICLE A small bone in the middle ear.

OUTER EAR The part of the ear containing the auditory canal.

PHARYNX A passageway from the mouth to the throat for air movement and food intake.

RESPIRATORY SYSTEM A system of organs that work together to make breathing possible, beginning with the nose and nasal passage and ending at the lungs.

RETINA The light-sensitive layer that lines the inside of the rear of the eyeball, which contains the rods and the cones for sight.

ROD A receptor cell in the retina of the eye that detects motion but no color.

SINUS A cavity (hollow space) such as that in the nose.

SKELETON The bony framework that supports the body and gives it shape.

VEINS Tubes that carry blood to the heart from different parts of the body.

VERTEBRAE Small, hollow bones making up the backbone that form a protective cover for the spinal cord.

FOR MORE INFORMATION

American Academy of Neurology (AAN)

201 Chicago Avenue

Minneapolis, MN 55415

(800) 879-1960

Website: www.aan.com

This organization facilitates the study and practice of neurologists, as well as protects neurologists by monitoring federal legislation. The AAN also advocates for neurology in the shaping of public policy.

American Academy of Ophthalmology

655 Beach Street

San Francisco, CA 94109

(415) 561-8500

Website: www.aao.org

This association of eye doctors aims to advance lifelong learning and study in the field of eye care and boasts a membership that comprises more than 90 percent of practicing eye doctors in the United States.

American Academy of Otolaryngology—Head and Neck Surgery

1650 Diagonal Road

Alexandria, VA 22314-2857

(703) 836-4444

Website: www.entnet.org

This organization represents doctors who specialize in treating the ear, nose, and throat as well as related areas of the head and neck.

American Association of Anatomists

9650 Rockville Pike

Bethesda, MD 20814-3998

(301) 634-7910

Website: www.anatomy.org

Founded in 1888 for the advancement of anatomical science, this organization promotes research, education, and professional development for members of this international community. Their members are mostly comprised of biomedical researchers and educators.

American Medical Association

AMA Plaza

330 N. Wabash Avenue

Chicago, IL 60611-5885

(800) 621-8335

Website: www.ama-assn.org

The goal of this member-driven organization is to promote the art and science of medicine and the betterment of public health. The organization also abides by a code of ethics and has thriving membership in every state in the United States.

American Psychiatric Association
1000 Wilson Boulevard, Suite 1825
Arlington, VA 22209
(888) 357-7924
Website: www.psychiatry.org
This member-driven organization is dedicated to ensuring the humane care and effective treatment of persons with mental disorders.

American Skin Association
6 East 43rd Street, 28th Floor
New York, NY 10017
(212) 889-4858
Website: www.americanskin.org
This group brings together medical professionals, research scientists, and patients and their families to promote skin health. Their mission is to advance research and drive public awareness about skin disease.

Canadian Ophthalmological Society
610-1525 Carling Avenue
Ottawa, ON K1Z 8R9
Canada

Canada

(613) 729-6779

Website: www.cos-sco.ca

This society represents eye physicians and surgeons in Canada and facilitates ongoing research and professional development for eye doctors.

Canadian Psychological Association

141 Laurier Avene West, Suite 702

Ottawa, ON K1P 5J3

Canada

(613) 237-2144

Website: www.cpa.ca

This professional organization represents the interests of psychology and attempts to promote clinical psychology in Canada.

Human Anatomy and Physiology Society

251 S. L. White Blvd.

P.O. Box 2945

La Grange, GA 30241-2945

Website: www.hapsweb.org

The Human Anatomy and Physiology Society is an educational organization with over 1,700 members teaching in high schools and universities in the United States and around the world. Among their goals is to promote quality human anatomy and physiology instruction, promote research, and organize professional development.

World Health Organization (WHO)

Avenue Appia 20

1211 Geneva 27

Switzerland

+ 41 22 791 21 11

Website: www.who.int

The World Health Organization works within the United Nations system on health matters, providing leadership in global health crises, shaping the direction of research, and setting standards for worldwide health organizations and policies. The WHO also provides technical support and monitoring to countries worldwide.

WEBSITES

Because of the changing nature of Internet links, Rosen Publishing has developed an online list of websites related to the subject of this book. This site is updated regularly. Please use this link to access this list:

http://www.rosenlinks.com/HB3D/Head

FOR FURTHER READING

Amsel, Sheri. *The Everything KIDS' Human Body Book: All You Need to Know About Your Body Systems From Head to Toe!* Avon, MA: Adams Media, 2012,

Biesty, Stephen and Richard Platt. *Stephen Biesty's Incredible Body.* New York, NY: Dorling Kindersley, 1998.

Burstein, John. *The Astounding Nervous System: How Does My Brain Work?* New York, NY: Crabtree Publishing Company, 2009.

Canavan, Thomas. *How Your Body Works: The Ultimate Illustrated Guide.* Mineola, NY: Dover Publications, 2015.

Carter, Rita. *The Human Brain Book.* New York, NY: DK Publishing, 2014.

Daniels, Patricia, Christina Wilsdon, and Jen Agresta. *Ultimate Bodypedia: An Amazing Inside-Out Tour of the Human Body.* Washington, DC: National Geographic Kids, 2014.

Green, John. *Human Anatomy in Full Color.* Mineola, NY: Dover Children's Science Books, 1996.

Human Body: A Visual Encyclopedia. New York, NY: DK Publishing, 2012.

Kapit, Wynn, and Lawrence M. Elson. *The Anatomy Coloring Book.* New York, NY: Pearson, 2013.

Macaulay, David. *The Way We Work: Getting to Know the Amazing Human Body.* New York, NY: HMH Books for Young Readers, 2008.

Page, Martyn. *Human Body: An Illustrated Guide to Every Part of the Human Body and How It Works.* New York, NY: DK Publishing, 2001.

Parker, Steve. *The Human Body Book* (Second Edition). New York, NY: DK ADULT, 2013.

Roberts, Alice. *The Complete Human Body* (Book & DVD-ROM). New York, NY: DK Publishing, 2010.

Rogers, Kara, editor. *Ear, Nose, and Throat.* New York, NY: Rosen Publishing, 2012.

Roza, Greg. *Inside the Human Body.* New York, NY: Rosen Publishing, 2007.

Simon, Seymour. *Bones.* New York, NY: HarperCollins, 2000.

Simon, Seymour. *The Brain: All About Our Nervous System and More!* New York, NY: HarperCollins, 2006.

Simon, Seymour. *Eyes and Ears.* New York, NY: HarperCollins, 2005.

Snedden, Robert. *Understanding the Brain and the Nervous System.* New York, NY: Rosen Publishing, 2010.

Stark, Freddy. *Start Exploring: Gray's Anatomy: A Fact-Filled Coloring Book.* Philadelphia, PA: Running Press Kids, 2011.

Stonehouse, Bernard, editor. *The Way Your Body Works.* London, England: Mitchell Beazley, 1974.

Taylor-Butler, Christine. *The Nervous System.* New York, NY: Children's Press, 2008.

Taylor-Butler, Christine. *The Respiratory System.* New York, NY: Children's Press, 2008.

White, Jon, editor. *How It Works Book of the Human Body* (Second Revised Edition). Single Issue Magazine, 2014.

INDEX

ABOUT THE AUTHORS

Jacintha Nathan is a retired nurse and an author with a particular interest in anatomy and physiology. She lives in Knoxville, Tennessee, with her husband, who is also a retired medical professional. This is her first book.

Walter Oleksy, who lives in Glenview, Illinois, is the author of over fifty books for young readers and adults, including *The Nervous System* and *The Circulatory System* for Rosen Publishing.

PHOTO CREDITS

Cover, p. 1 (head) © iStockphoto.com/Eraxion; cover, p. 1 (hand) © iStockphoto.com/Nixxphotography;pp. 5, 12 3D4Medical/Science Source; pp. 9, 38–39 MediaForMedical/UIG/Getty Images; pp. 10–11, 13, 40–41 BSIP/UIG/Getty Images; p. 15 Leonello Calvetti/Stocktrek Images/Getty Images; p. 17 Nicholas Mayeux/Stocktrek Images/Getty Images; pp. 18–19, 22–23, 49 © SuperStock, Inc.; pp. 20, 28, 46, 47 SCIEPRO/Science Photo Library/Getty Images; pp. 24–25 Science Picture Co/Science Source; p. 27 Alan Gesek/Stocktrek Images/Getty Images; p. 31, 32–33, 34 Sebastian Kaulitzki/Science Photo Library/Getty Images; p. 37 Sophie Jacopin/Science Source; p. 42 Claus Lunau/Science Source; p. 44 Encyclopaedia Britannica/UIG/Getty Images; pp. 50–51 Anatomical Travelogue/Science Source/Getty Images; back cover (figure) © iStockphoto.com/comotion design; cover and interior pages graphic elements © iStockphoto.com/StudioM1, wenani/Shutterstock.com, Egor Tetiushev/Shutterstock.com.

Designer: Brian Garvey; Editor: Tracey Baptiste
Photo Researcher: Karen Huang